DENTAL HEALTH

COOKBOOK

Fun ways and Nutritious Recipes to Keep Teeth and Mouth Healthy!

With Meal plan bonus

LOUIS M. MADSEN

TABLE OF CONTENT

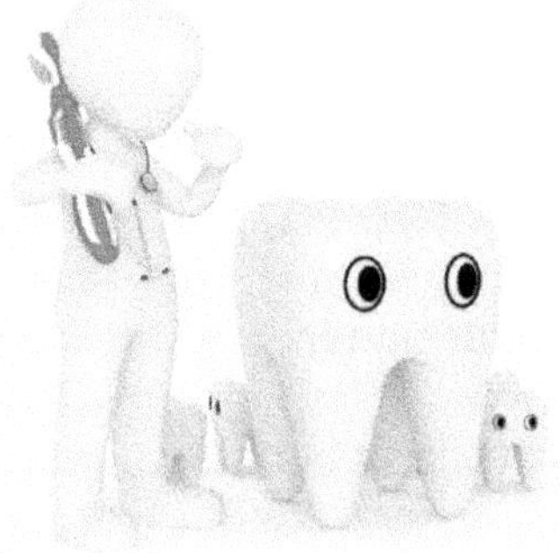

INTRODUCTION TO DENTAL HEALTH

Question:

Did you know that according to the journal of dental researches, about 2.4 billion people worldwide have tooth problems as you read this article? Sadly, by the end of this year, another 190 million people will be included in this endless list of people with tooth problems. The question then becomes: 'Why? Why is it that so many people have tooth-related problems?'

The Answer!

Well, it has been in observation since over the years till this present age that people do not realize how significant it is for them to put in (more) efforts to treat and maintain their oral health, they rather spend their last dime to examine any fault in the other parts of their bodies thereby having an unbalanced body improvement rather than a properly balanced one. It is as well important to care for the health orally.

WHAT IS ORAL HEALTH?

Let's define Health

According to World Health Organization, health is defined as, 'a state of complete physical, mental & social well-being & not merely the absence of disease & infirmity'.

Now What is Oral Health?

Oral health is the health of the mouth, including the teeth, gums, tongue, and other structures in the mouth. Good oral hygiene is important for overall health and can help prevent tooth decay, gum disease, and other health problems.

The ultimate goal of dental care is good oral health, it is my concern to impact a positive oral health knowledge and nutrition. The Mouth is the door to castle called body. So people should have their healthy oral cavity and should have a proper knowledge about it.

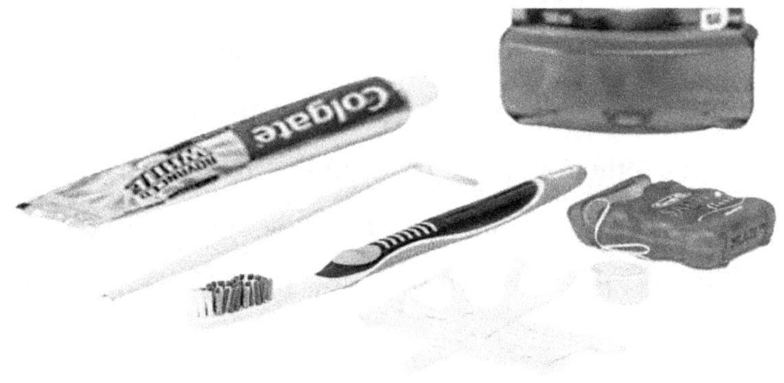

Steeve was a man who had always been embarrassed of his teeth. He had not gone to the dentist for his regular check-ups, leading to years of poor oral health. Steeve was constantly in pain and had a hard time eating or speaking without feeling discomfort.

One day, Steeve went to the dentist, and the doctor gave them a stern lecture about the importance of taking care of his teeth. The doctor advised them to ensure he brushed and flossed twice a day and to have him avoid sugary and acidic foods.

Steeve however is always tempted to eat sugary foods but that all changed when he came across one of my social media post about how to reverse dental condition then he click on the link to get the book, he was motivated to follow the instructions and started to make changes to his diet. He cut out sugary and acidic foods and drinks, and began to eat more fruits, vegetables, and whole grains. He also started to brush and floss twice daily, and even use mouthwash.

Within a few weeks, Steeve's teeth were looking and feeling much better. He was no longer in pain, and was able to eat and speak without any discomfort. Steeve was so proud of himself for making the decision to take care of his health.

Steeve soon began to made sure to keep up with his oral hygiene routine, ensuring his teeth stayed healthy and strong. He was thankful for the changes he had made, and was proud to show off his beautiful smile. He had reversed his poor oral health with the right diet and dental care routine. He was determined to keep up his healthy habits, so he could always have a bright and beautiful smile.

Dental health is a vital part of overall health and wellbeing Knowing about the importance of good dental hygiene habits can help them maintain their teeth and gums for a lifetime. Good dental hygiene starts with brushing teeth twice a day, flossing once a day, and visiting the dentist for regular checkups. Brushing removes plaque, a sticky film of bacteria, from the surfaces of teeth. Flossing removes plaque and food particles from between teeth, where toothbrush bristles can't reach.

In addition to brushing and flossing, People should limit their intake of sugary foods and drinks because it can contribute to tooth decay. People also avoid eating sticky, chewy foods, such as gummy candies, as these can get stuck between teeth and cause cavities.

Regular checkups with a dentist are also important for dental health. During a checkup, the dentist will clean teeth and check for cavities and gum disease. By knowing about the importance of good dental hygiene and visiting the dentist regularly, healthy teeth and gums can be maintained for a lifetime.

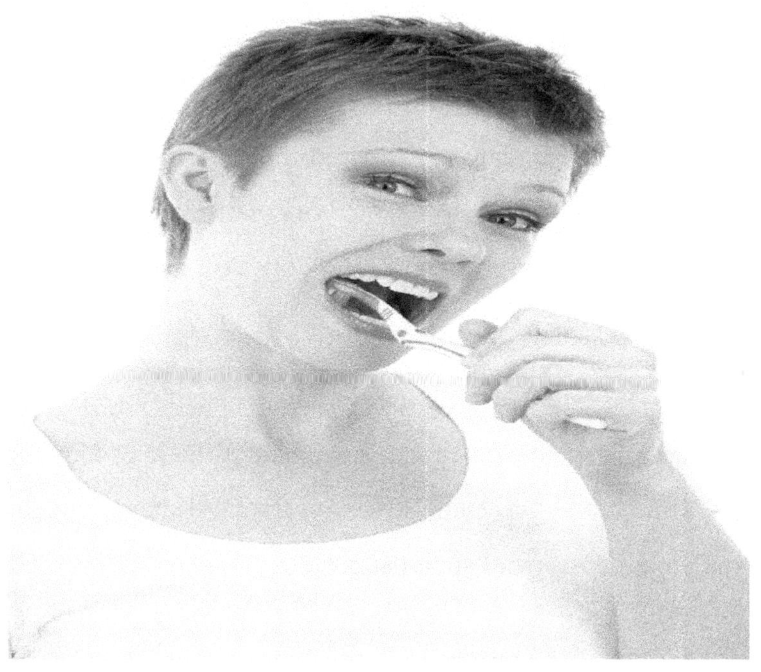

CHAPTER 1

THE BENEFITS OF GOOD ORAL HEALTH

Good oral health is vital for general health and wellbeing. Regular dental care and healthy habits can help prevent tooth decay, cavities, gum disease, and other related diseases. Maintaining good oral health can have a positive impact on your quality of life in many ways.

1. Improved Appearance: Having healthy teeth and a bright smile can help you feel more confident in your appearance, which can lead to improved self-esteem and also can have a big impact on your overall appearance. Taking care of your teeth can help you look and feel more attractive.

2. Improved Self-Confidence: Having a healthy teeth and gums can boost your self-esteem and confidence. Having healthy teeth and gums can give you the confidence to take on new challenges and social situations.

3. Better Overall Health: Poor oral health has been linked to many serious health conditions, such as heart disease, stroke, and diabetes. Brushing and flossing regularly can help reduce your risk of these and other serious health issues.

4. Reduced risk for other health problems: Poor oral hygiene can lead to the development of cavities and gum disease, which can have a negative impact on your overall health. Good oral hygiene can help reduce your risk of developing these problems.

5. Reduced Pain and Discomfort: Tooth decay, gum disease, and other oral health conditions can cause pain and discomfort. Taking good care of your teeth can help prevent or reduce these issues.

7. Improved Quality of Life: Taking care of your teeth and gums can help improve your overall quality of life. Having healthy teeth and gums can make it easier to eat, speak, and socialize with confidence.

8. Better nutrition: Healthy teeth and gums allow you to chew and digest food more effectively, which can help you get the nutrients you need to stay healthy.

9. Improved social life: Good oral hygiene can help you make a good first impression with others, which can lead to more successful social interactions.

10. Promote Aesthetic Value: Healthy teeth, gums, smile and overall oral hygiene contribute to the attractiveness of your face and enhance your facial aesthetics.

Therefore, Overall health and well-being can be determined by Good Oral Health. Taking steps to maintain healthy teeth and gums can help you enjoy a lifetime of good oral health.

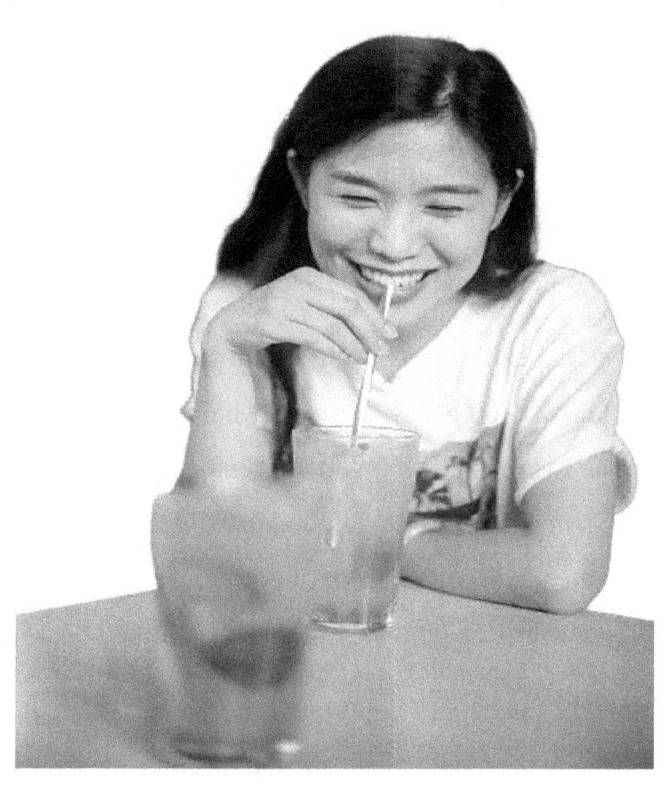

CHAPTER 2

Understanding the Relationship between Nutrition and Dental Health

Dental health and nutrition go hand in hand in order to achieve and maintain good oral health. Nutrition is important to dental health because it provides the essential vitamins and minerals that help teeth and gums stay strong and healthy. Eating a balanced diet that is low in sugar and high in nutrient-rich foods, such as fruits and vegetables, whole grains, and lean proteins can help protect your teeth and gums against cavities and gum disease, prevent tooth decay and other dental problems.

Good dental health starts with brushing and flossing your teeth at least twice a day. Brushing helps remove bacteria and plaque that can build up on the teeth and cause cavities, while flossing helps remove food particles that get stuck between the teeth. It is also important to visit a dentist regularly for professional cleanings and routine check-ups.

Nutrition is also an important part of dental health. Nutrition plays a major role in maintaining proper dental health. Eating a balanced diet that is low in sugar and high in nutrient-rich foods, such as fruits and vegetables, can help protect your teeth and gums against cavities and gum disease as these types of foods are major contributors to dental plaque. Additionally, foods that are high in calcium and phosphorus, such as dairy products, can help strengthen teeth and promote healthy gums, and prevent decay.

Nutrient-rich foods can help strengthen teeth and protect them from bacteria and decay. Calcium, phosphorus, and vitamin D are all essential for healthy, strong teeth. Foods like milk, cheese, yogurt, and green leafy vegetables are all good sources of these nutrients. Eating crunchy fruits and vegetables can also help clean the teeth and gums and keep bacteria from accumulating. Additionally, consuming foods that are high in fiber can help reduce the risk of gum disease. Eating enough of these foods can help keep teeth and gums healthy, and reduce the risk of cavities and gum disease.

It is also important to limit the amount of sugary and starchy snacks you eat. These types of foods can lead to tooth decay and gum disease if consumed in excess. This is because these types of foods contain bacteria that feed on the sugar and produce acids that damage teeth. Eating too many of these foods can lead to cavities, gum disease, and other dental problems.

It is also very important to stay hydrated by drinking a lot of water throughout the day. This can help rinse away food particles and bacteria that can build up on the teeth. Drinking plenty of water can also help keep the mouth hydrated, which can help reduce the risk of cavities. Staying hydrated also helps prevent dry mouth, which can lead to bad breath and other oral health issues. Other beverages that contain sugar, such as juice and soda, should be avoided as they can contribute to tooth decay and gum disease.

In addition to eating a balanced diet, it is important to practice good oral hygiene. Brushing and flossing regularly can help remove plaque and food particles from the teeth and gums and reduce the risk of cavities and gum disease.

Overall, dental health and nutrition go hand in hand in order to maintain good oral health. Eating a balanced diet, brushing and flossing regularly, and visiting your dentist regularly are all important components of maintaining good dental health, practicing good oral hygiene can help keep teeth and gums strong and decrease the risk of dental problems.

In conclusion, nutrition and dental health are closely linked. Eating a balanced diet and practicing good oral hygiene can help reduce the risk of cavities and gum disease. By following these steps, you can help ensure that your teeth and gums stay healthy and strong for many years to come.

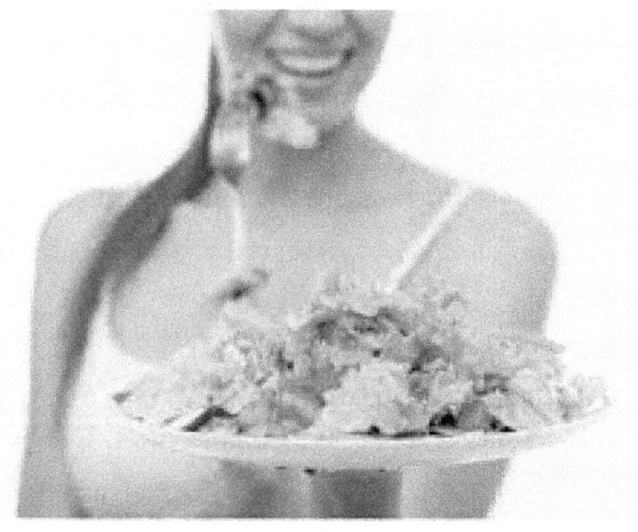

CHAPTER 3

Dietary Strategies to Promote Dental Health

1. Eat a Diet High in Nutrient-rich Foods: Eating a diet that is rich in nutrient-dense foods such as fruits, vegetables, and whole grains can help promote dental health. These foods are packed with essential vitamins and minerals that help build strong, healthy teeth.

2. Avoid Sugary and Acidic Foods: Sugary and acidic foods can cause tooth decay and cavities. It is best to avoid these foods as much as possible, as they can do more harm than good to your dental health. Foods and drinks that are high in acid, such as citrus fruits, can erode tooth enamel. Try to limit how often these are consumed.

3. Choose Low-sugar Beverages: Sugary beverages such as soda, sweetened juices, and energy drinks can harm teeth if consumed in excess. Drinking water, milk, unsweetened tea or coffee instead is a better choice.

4. Consume Dairy Products: Dairy products such as milk, yogurt, and cheese are high in calcium, which helps to strengthen teeth and prevent cavities.

5. Eat Crunchy Fruits and Vegetables: Crunchy fruits and vegetables act like a natural toothbrush and help to remove plaque and debris from the teeth such as apples, carrots, and celery, help to naturally clean teeth and promote saliva production.

6. Snack Smartly: If you are craving a snack, try to reach for a healthy option such as nuts, seeds, or sugar-free gum. Choose snacks that are low in sugar and starches, such as fresh fruits, vegetables, cheese, and yogurt.

7. Chew Sugar-free Gum: Chewing sugar-free gum for at least 20 minutes after eating can help to reduce the amount of acid and bacteria in the mouth and promote dental health.

8. Avoid sticky foods: Sticky foods, such as dried fruit and candy, can stick to teeth and increase the risk of cavities.

9. Floss regularly: Flossing removes food particles and plaque from between teeth that a toothbrush cannot reach. It should be done at least once a day.

10. Use fluoridated toothpaste: Fluoridated toothpaste helps to prevent cavities. Make sure to use a toothpaste that has the Dental Association seal of approval.

11. Follow a Regular Oral Hygiene Routine: Brushing your teeth twice a day and flossing at least once a day is essential for maintaining good dental health. Additionally, make sure to visit your dentist for regular check-ups and cleanings.

Following these dietary strategies can help to promote good dental health and ensure that your teeth and gums stay healthy for years to come.

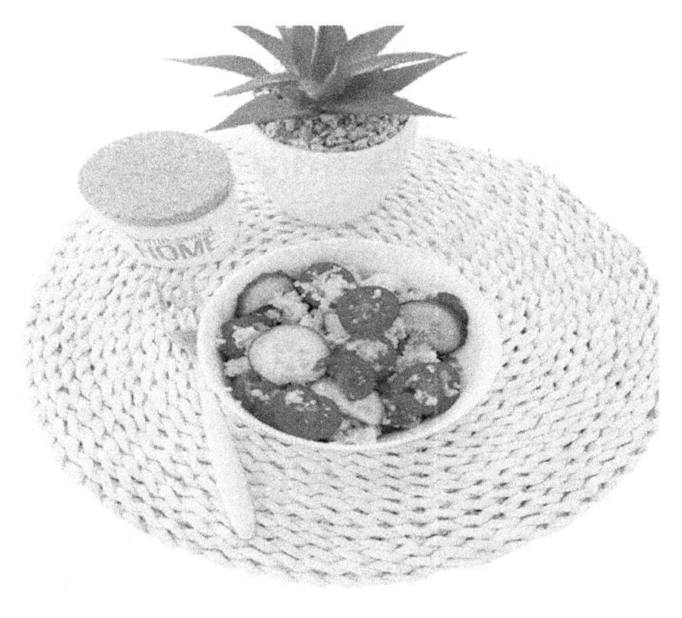

CHAPTER 4

HEALTHY DENTAL SNACK IDEAS

1. Unsweetened plain popcorn

Unsweetened plain popcorn is an excellent choice of healthy dental snack. Popcorn is a whole grain, making it a nutritious snack that is low in calories, fat and sugar. It also contains dietary fiber, which helps promote good oral health by providing a source of essential nutrients and keeping the mouth clean. Popcorn is a crunchy snack, which helps to break up plaque and food particles, reducing the risk of cavities and other dental problems. Additionally, popcorn is a low-acid snack, which helps to balance the amount of acid in the mouth, further reducing the risk of tooth decay.

Therefore, unsweetened plain popcorn can be a great choice for those looking for a healthy snack that promotes dental health. It is a good choice for those trying to maintain a healthy diet and a healthy mouth, and it can even be enjoyed as a snack during movie nights or family gatherings.

2. Celery sticks with natural peanut butter

Celery sticks with natural peanut butter are a healthy dental snack idea! The celery sticks are crunchy, which helps remove plaque and food particles from teeth. The natural peanut butter provides a healthy source of protein that helps your body build strong teeth and bones. Plus, the peanut butter has a delicious flavor that will satisfy your sweet tooth without any added sugar. Enjoy this snack without worrying about cavities or other dental problems!

This snack is also a great option for those with sensitive teeth. The natural peanut butter does not contain any added sugar, which means it won't irritate your sensitive teeth. Plus, the celery sticks provide a crunchy texture that won't aggravate your teeth. Enjoy this snack knowing that it's good for your oral health!

This snack is also easy to prepare and can be enjoyed on the go. Just grab some celery sticks and natural peanut butter and you're good to go! Enjoy this healthy dental snack anytime, anywhere. So, if you're looking for a healthy and tasty snack, try celery sticks with natural peanut butter! This snack is sure to please your taste buds while also keeping your teeth healthy. Enjoy!

3. Unsweetened plain yogurt with fresh berries

Unsweetened plain yogurt with fresh berries is a great healthy dental snack idea. The yogurt helps to replenish the good bacteria in your mouth while the fresh berries are a great source of Vitamin C, which helps to keep your gums healthy. The yogurt also helps to neutralize the acids that can cause damage to teeth. Furthermore, the combination of the yogurt and berries is a great way to satisfy your sweet tooth without the added sugar that can cause dental problems. This snack is low in calories and packed with beneficial nutrients, making it an ideal choice for those looking to take better care of their teeth.

In conclusion, unsweetened plain yogurt with fresh berries is a great healthy dental snack idea. This snack is low in calories and packed with beneficial nutrients that can help keep your teeth and gums healthy. Plus, it's an easy and delicious way to satisfy your sweet tooth without the added sugar.

So, if you're looking for a healthy dental snack, give unsweetened plain yogurt with fresh berries a try. Your teeth will thank you!

4. Apple slices with plain Greek yogurt dip

Apple slices with plain Greek yogurt dip make an ideal healthy dental snack especially for kids. The crunchiness of the apple slices helps to clean the teeth, while the calcium and probiotics in the yogurt help to promote healthy gums and teeth. This snack is low in sugar and provides a boost of protein and other essential vitamins and minerals. Plus, the yogurt dip adds a bit of sweetness without the added sugar. This snack is sure to put a smile on your face.

This snack is easy to make and is sure to become a family favorite. Simply cut up some apple slices and put them in a bowl. Mix together some plain Greek yogurt and a bit of honey or maple syrup, if desired. Serve the dip alongside the apple slices. Enjoy!

5. Nuts, such as almonds, walnuts, and cashews

Nuts, like almonds, walnuts, and cashews, are an excellent choice for a healthy dental snack. They are packed with important vitamins and minerals that help to support healthy teeth and gums. Plus, the crunchy texture of the nuts can help to scrub away food particles and plaque.

Almonds are an especially good choice for dental health because they are high in calcium and contain a compound that helps to reduce inflammation. Walnuts are also an excellent snack for dental health because they are high in omega-3 fatty acids, which have anti-inflammatory properties. Cashews are high in phosphorus, which helps to strengthen tooth enamel. Eating a handful of nuts a few times a week is a great way to support your oral health.

In addition to the nutritional benefits of nuts, they also provide a flavorful and satisfying snack. You can mix and match different types of nuts or even add other dried fruits to create a delicious and healthy snack that's perfect for your teeth.

Nuts are a great snack for both adults and children, so they're the perfect choice for a dental-friendly snack!

6. Carrot and cucumber sticks with hummus

Carrot and cucumber sticks with hummus make for a great healthy dental snack idea. The crunchy texture of the carrots and cucumbers helps to scrub away plaque and bacteria from the surface of teeth, while the hummus is a good source of calcium, which helps to strengthen teeth and bones. Additionally, the hummus contains healthy fats that can help to keep the gums healthy and strong. Finally, the combination of ingredients makes for a tasty, nutritious snack that can boost overall dental health.

This snack is great for people of all ages and can be enjoyed as part of a larger healthy meal. Carrot and cucumber sticks can easily be cut up and served with hummus, making it a convenient snack that can be taken on the go. It is also a great option for those with dietary restrictions, as it is gluten-free, dairy-free, and vegan-friendly.

Overall, carrot and cucumber sticks with hummus make for a tasty, nutritious, and dental-friendly snack that can be enjoyed by people of all ages. It is a great way to boost overall dental health and can be easily taken on the go.

Happy snacking!

7. Hard-boiled eggs

Hard-boiled eggs make the perfect healthy dental snack. They are packed with essential vitamins and minerals, such as protein, calcium, and phosphorus, that help strengthen teeth and bones. Plus, the crunchy texture of eggs helps scrub away plaque and food particles, making them a great snack choice for dental health. Eating eggs can also help reduce the risk of developing cavities, as the protein helps to stimulate saliva production, which helps to balance the pH levels in the mouth. Eggs also contain lutein, which may help protect teeth from erosion from acidic foods.

With all these benefits and more, hard-boiled eggs are an excellent snack for healthy teeth and gums.

In addition to being packed with dental health benefits, hard-boiled eggs are also incredibly easy to make. All you need to do is place your eggs in a pot, fill it with cold water, and bring it to a boil. Once boiled, you can let the eggs cool down and they are ready to eat. Hard-boiled eggs make a great snack on the go, as they can be peeled and eaten right away. Plus, they can be added to salads, sandwiches, or enjoyed alone for a quick and healthy snack.

With all their dental health benefits, hard-boiled eggs are an excellent snack idea. Not only are they packed with essential vitamins and minerals, but they are also incredibly easy to make and can be enjoyed as a quick and healthy snack on the go. So if you're looking for a snack that is great for your teeth, try adding hard-boiled eggs to your daily routine.

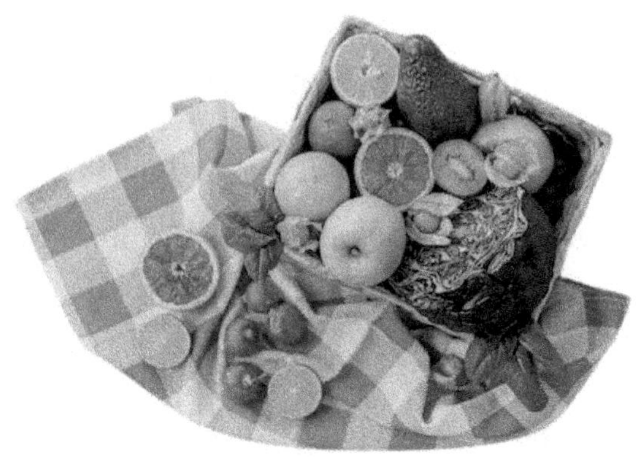

Other Healthy Dental Snack Ideas

    i.   Baked kale chips

    ii.   Edamame

    iii.   Avocado toast with fresh tomato slices

    iv.   Cottage cheese with fresh fruit

    v.   Plain rice cakes with nut butter

    vi.   Roasted chickpeas

    vii.   Pumpkin seeds

    viii.   Grilled salmon with steamed vegetables

    ix.   Air-popped popcorn with a sprinkle of cinnamon

    x.   Sliced bell peppers with guacamole

    xi.   Banana with almond butter

    xii.   Celery with almond butter

    xiii.   Whole grain crackers with cheese

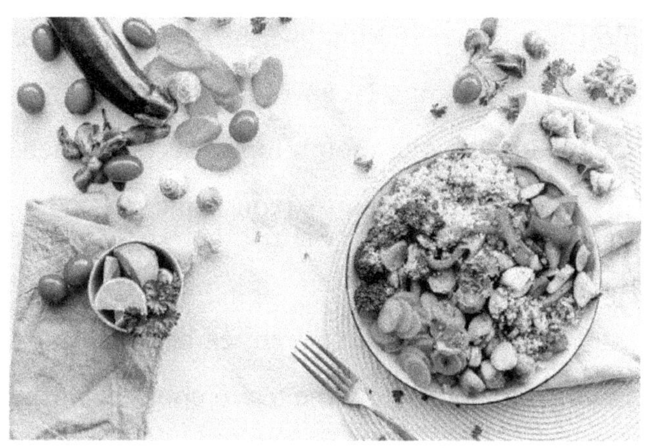

CHAPTER 5

RECIPES FOR DENTAL HEALTH

1. Coconut Oil Pulling: Melt 1 tablespoon of coconut oil in a microwave-safe container. Swish the oil around your mouth for 10-20 minutes, then spit it out. The oil will help to reduce inflammation, remove bacteria, and whiten teeth.

2. Homemade Toothpaste: Mix together 1 tablespoon of baking soda, 1 teaspoon of hydrogen peroxide, and 1 teaspoon of sea salt. Add a few drops of peppermint essential oil to give it a fresh taste. Brush your teeth with this mixture twice a day to reduce plaque, whiten teeth and freshen breath.

3. Apple Cider Vinegar Mouthwash: Mix 1 tablespoon of apple cider vinegar into 1 cup of warm water. Swish the combination around your mouth for 30 seconds, then spit it out. This mouthwash helps to reduce plaque and freshen breath.

4. Green Tea Rinse: Steep 1 green tea bag in 1 cup of hot water for 10 minutes. Allow the tea to cool, then use it as a mouth rinse. The antioxidants in green tea can help to reduce inflammation and protect against oral bacteria.

5. Aloe Vera Gel: Apply a small amount of aloe Vera gel to your toothbrush and brush your teeth with it. Aloe Vera helps to reduce inflammation and fight against tooth decay.

6. Lemon Rinse: Squeeze the juice of 1 lemon into 1 cup of water and swish it around your mouth for 30 seconds. Spit it out and rinse with ordinary water. The citric acid in lemons helps to whiten teeth and reduce plaque.

7. Turmeric Toothpaste: Mix together 1 tablespoon of turmeric powder, 1 teaspoon of coconut oil, and 1 teaspoon of baking soda. Brush your teeth with this mixture twice a day to reduce inflammation and fight against gum disease.

8. Activated Charcoal Rinse: Swish 1 teaspoon of activated charcoal powder in 1 cup of water for 1 minute. Spit it out, then rinse with ordinary water. This rinse helps to remove toxins and reduce plaque.

9. Baking Soda Mouthwash: Mix together 1 teaspoon of baking soda and 1 cup of water. Swish the combination around your mouth for 30 seconds, then spit it out. Baking soda helps to reduce plaque and freshen breath.

10. Herbal Teas: Drink herbal teas that are high in antioxidants, such as green tea or chamomile tea. The antioxidants can help to reduce inflammation and fight against oral bacteria.

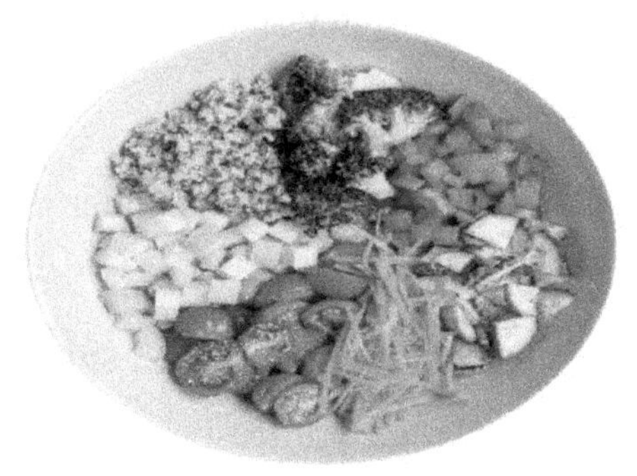

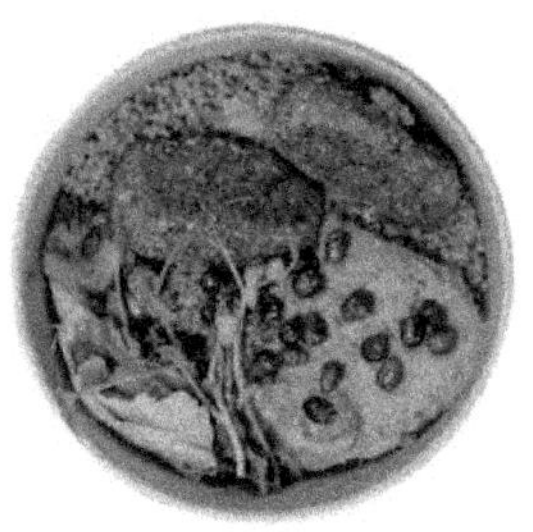

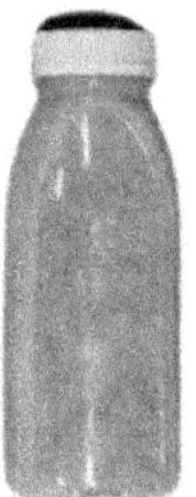

MEAL PLAN BONUS

Breakfast Recipes

1.Oatmeal with Berries: Start your day off with a healthy and delicious breakfast! This oatmeal dish is packed with essential vitamins and minerals that promote dental health. Start by cooking the oatmeal following the package guidelines. Top with your favorite berries like blueberries, strawberries, raspberries, and blackberries. Add a dash of cinnamon and a sprinkle of honey for extra flavor.

2.Smoothie Bowl: Create a delicious breakfast smoothie bowl that is rich in vitamins and minerals that are great for your dental health. Start by blending your favorite fruits like bananas, strawberries, blueberries, and raspberries. Add a handful of spinach or kale for an additional nutritional enhancement. Pour the smoothie into a bowl and top with your favorite nuts and seeds like almonds, walnuts, and chia seeds.

3.Yogurt Parfait: Start your day off with a yogurt parfait that is rich in probiotics, which can help promote healthy teeth and gums. Layer yogurt with your favorite fruits, nuts, and seeds. Top with a pinch of cinnamon for an additional flavor.

4.Avocado Toast: Toast whole-wheat bread and top with mashed avocado for a tasty and dental-friendly breakfast. The healthy fats from the avocado are great for promoting dental health. Add a sprinkle of sea salt and a squeeze of lemon juice for added flavor.

5.Egg and Vegetable Scramble: Start your morning with a nutrient-packed egg and vegetable scramble. Start by scrambling eggs in a pan with your favorite vegetables like bell peppers, tomatoes, mushrooms, and spinach. Add a sprinkle of cheddar cheese for extra flavor. Serve with some whole-grain toast for a complete breakfast.

No matter what breakfast you choose, it's important to remember that a healthy and balanced diet is essential for good dental health. Eating plenty of fruits, vegetables, and whole grains can help keep your teeth and gums healthy and strong.

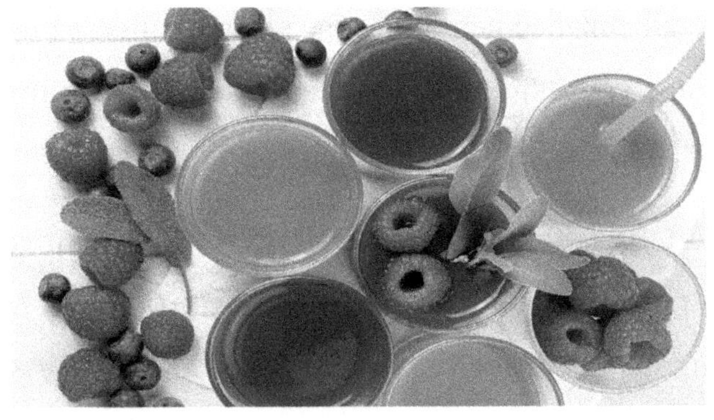

Lunch Recipes

1. Grilled Salmon with Broccoli and Brown Rice: Grilled salmon is an excellent source of protein and omega-3 fatty acids, which are beneficial for dental health. This meal also contains calcium-rich broccoli and whole grain brown rice to increase the nutritional value.

2. Lentil Soup with Whole Wheat Toast: Lentils are high in fiber and contain folate, a vitamin important for tooth health. Serve this soup with some whole wheat toast for an added crunch.

3. Turkey Wrap with Spinach and Avocado: Lean turkey is a great source of protein and contains phosphorus, an essential mineral for tooth enamel. Wrapping it up with some spinach and avocado adds an extra dose of vitamins and minerals.

4. Quinoa Salad with Veggies: Quinoa is a great source of fiber and is high in phosphorus, which helps keep teeth strong. Topped with colorful vegetables and a light vinaigrette, this salad makes for a delicious and nutritious meal.

5. Greek Yogurt Parfait: Greek yogurt is packed with calcium, which helps keep teeth and bones healthy. Layer it with some fresh fruit and your favorite granola for a tasty, tooth-friendly treat.

6. Hummus and Veggie Sandwich: Hummus is a great source of protein and contains vitamins and minerals that are important for dental health. Serve on whole wheat bread with your favorite vegetables for a delicious and nutritious sandwich.

7. PB&J Smoothie: Peanut butter is full of protein, calcium and phosphorus, which are all important for keeping teeth strong. Blend it with frozen berries, banana and a little almond milk for a healthy and delicious smoothie.

8. Apple with Cheese: Apples are loaded with fiber and vitamin C, which are both beneficial for dental health. Pair with a slice of cheese for added calcium and protein.

9. Kale and Avocado Salad: Kale is packed with vitamins and minerals that are great for dental health. Add avocado to increase the protein and healthy fats. Top with a light vinaigrette for a tasty and nutritious lunch.

10. Grilled Chicken Wrap: Grilled chicken is a great source of protein and is low in fat. Wrap it up in a whole wheat wrap with some lettuce, tomato and avocado for a delicious and tooth-friendly meal.

By including these tooth-friendly lunch recipes in your weekly meal plan, you can ensure that your dental health stays in tip-top shape. Bon Appetit!

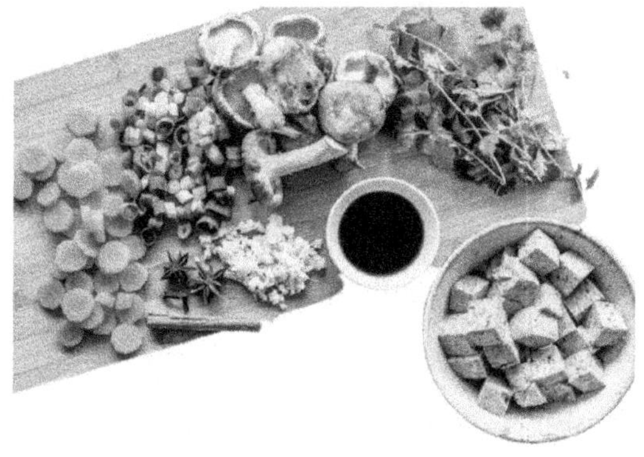

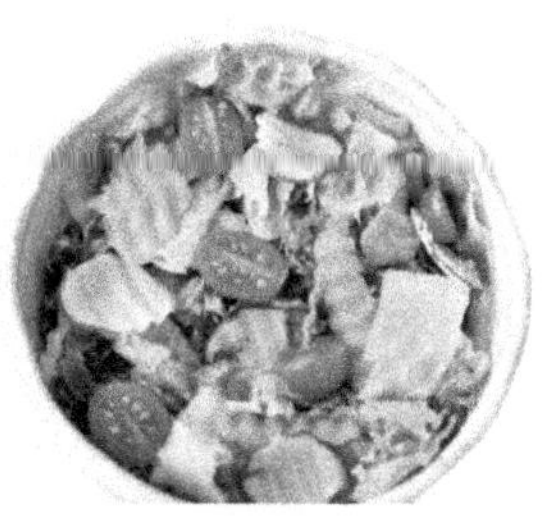

Dinner Recipes

1. Avocado & Salmon Salad: Start by combining diced avocado, cubed cooked salmon, and sliced cucumber in a bowl. Top with a light vinaigrette and a sprinkle of fresh lemon juice.

2. Grilled Veggie Skewers: Skewer a variety of vegetables, such as bell peppers, mushrooms, and onion. Grill until lightly charred and serve over a bed of quinoa or brown rice.

3. Baked Salmon with Herbs & Garlic: Rub a salmon fillet with olive oil, garlic, rosemary, and thyme. Then leave in the oven for 15minutes to Bake, or until thoroughly cooked. Serve along with a side of roasted vegetables.

4. Zucchini Noodle Bowl: Spiralize zucchini and combine with a light vinaigrette. Add cooked shrimp, cherry tomatoes, and feta cheese.

5. Roasted Cauliflower & Broccoli: Roast cauliflower and broccoli florets in the oven with garlic, olive oil, salt, and pepper. Serve with a squeeze of lemon juice and some freshly grated Parmesan cheese.

6. Kale & Quinoa Salad: Combine cooked quinoa, kale, feta cheese, cherry tomatoes, and toasted almonds. Top with a light vinaigrette and a sprinkle of fresh lemon juice.

7. Lentil & Spinach Stew: Saute onion, garlic, and carrots in olive oil. Add canned tomatoes and cooked lentils. Simmer for 15 minutes, then add fresh spinach and cook for another 5 minutes. Serve with a splotch of Greek yogurt.

8. Baked Sweet Potato Fries: Cut sweet potatoes into wedges and place on a baking sheet. Sprinkle with some olive oil and spice with pepper and salt. Bake in the oven till it turns golden and crispy.

9. Coconut Curry Soup: Saute onion, garlic, and ginger in a pot. Add some curry powder, with diced tomatoes, and coconut milk. Simmer for 15 minutes, then add cooked chickpeas and cooked quinoa.

10. Grilled Chicken & Vegetable Wrap: Grill chicken and vegetables. Serve in a wrap with hummus and Greek yogurt.

11. Quinoa & Vegetable Bowl: Cook quinoa according to package instructions. Top with roasted vegetables, feta cheese, and a light vinaigrett

CONCLUSION

Continuing to Promote Good Dental Health

Based on the evidence provided, it can be concluded that continuing to promote good dental health is important for overall health and well-being. Good dental health can help prevent a variety of health conditions and diseases, as well as reduce the risk of oral cancer. Additionally, good oral hygiene can improve overall quality of life and boost confidence. Therefore, it is important to continue to promote good dental health in order to maintain optimal health and wellbeing.

By encouraging proper oral hygiene, such as brushing and flossing twice daily, scheduling regular dental checkups, and avoiding sugary and acidic foods and drinks, individuals can protect their dental health and overall health. Education and awareness are key when it comes to promoting good dental health and preventing oral and other health issues. Therefore, it is important to continue to educate people about proper oral hygiene and the importance of maintaining good dental health.

Overall, continuing to promote good dental health is important for overall health and well-being. Therefore, it is important to continue to raise awareness about the importance of good oral hygiene and the impact it can have on overall health.

Good oral health can have a positive impact on your overall health and wellbeing, so it is important to take steps to ensure that your mouth is healthy and free from dental problems.

www.ingramcontent.com/pod-product-compliance
Lightning Source LLC
Chambersburg PA
CBHW072342270726
48659CB00023B/2263